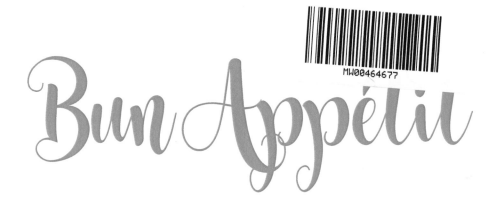

Bun Appétit

A Simple Guide
to Eating Right
During Pregnancy

By **TOREY ARMUL**

MS, RD, CSSD

This book is dedicated to my three boys:
Scott, thank you for your endless encouragement, love and
proofreading skills. Thank you, Brady, for sitting on my lap,
typing (banging) on the keyboard and keeping me company
while I wrote. And to our newest baby boy arriving in February,
thank you for being the fire in my belly (literally) and the real
inspiration behind this book.

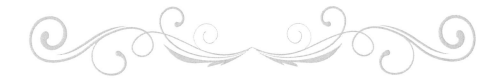

Table of Contents

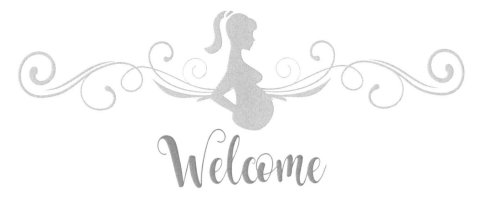

Welcome

So you've got a bun in the oven? Congratulations! Now what should be *in* your kitchen oven?

This book shares what foods to eat during pregnancy - and when to eat them - to coincide with your baby's growth and development each trimester.

You've heard the phrase, "You are what you eat." I believe, "You are *and your baby is* what you eat." And when you eat it! As you'll read in each chapter, your baby relies on the right nutrients at the right times for optimal growth and development.

You may be asking yourself, "Does it *really* matter what I eat?"

I'm a registered dietitian, and I asked myself that question multiple times during my first pregnancy. No judgment here! The more I've learned over the years and the latest research on prenatal nutrition has answered my question with a resounding "yes." Let me share this information so you'll reach the same conclusion, too.

Over the next 40 weeks, your baby will grow from a microscopic seedling to a wriggling, full-term baby. He or she will grow five vital organs — a heart, a liver, a brain, lungs and kidneys — and an entire skeletal system, circulatory system, digestive system and reproductive system. This extraordinary feat relies on well-functioning stem cells, oxygen-rich blood and proper DNA production, all of which are influenced by the nutrients in your food.

By eating the right foods during the right stage of development, you'll help give your baby what he or she needs, when he or she needs it. Failing to do so has serious and long-term consequences according to the Academy of Nutrition and Dietetics:

"Inadequate levels of key nutrients during crucial periods of fetal development may lead to reprogramming within fetal tissues, predisposing the infant to chronic conditions in later life. Those conditions include obesity, cardiovascular disease, bone health, cognition, immune function, and diabetes."

It's a frightening thought, but there is good news: You don't have to eat perfectly during pregnancy. Mother Nature has the situation covered, somewhat. She's designed it so that baby takes priority and usually gets what he or she needs from mom. Unfortunately, this can be to the detriment of the mother's own health.

While your focus is on your growing baby (and understandably so!), know that it's equally important for you to be eating well for your own health.

Feeding your body the right way can better prepare you for the evolving demands of motherhood: labor and childbirth, breastfeeding, caring for a newborn and potential future pregnancies.

So yes, it does matter what you eat during pregnancy, both for your health and the health of your growing baby. You and your baby are inseparable during pregnancy, a single unit connected in the deepest way. It's no surprise, then, that a healthier mom makes a healthier baby. What you do, your baby does. Where you go, your baby goes. What you eat, your baby eats.

What Should You Eat?

Let me start by saying that it does not have to be perfect. Women are granted considerable leniency to deal with the various food challenges of pregnancy: exhaustion, all-day morning sickness, smell and taste changes and comfort food cravings.

Do your best. Make an honest effort to eat well (this book will help!) and don't use pregnancy as a 10-month-long excuse for eating junk food. Believe me, that excuse doesn't end with pregnancy. It grows louder as your life gets even busier and "me time" dwindles. "I can eat this because I'm pregnant" evolves into "because I'm breastfeeding," "because there's no time for grocery shopping," "because I'm exhausted" and so on.

Your baby and children will give you a permanent excuse to eat unhealthy foods. Try to reshape that thought now, during pregnancy. Your children should not be your reason to be unhealthy. They're one of your greatest reasons to be healthy!

Why You Need a Prenatal Vitamin

Babies need a wide variety of nutrients throughout pregnancy, so it's a good idea to follow a basic healthy eating pattern with

- ☑ plenty of fruits and vegetables
- ☑ lean proteins
- ☑ whole grains
- ☑ healthy fats

A prenatal vitamin is also essential for filling nutritional gaps and meeting the increased demand for certain nutrients during pregnancy. Many experts believe that even a nutritious diet won't supply enough iron or folate to meet a pregnant woman's needs, so supplementation may be necessary.

Can't stomach your prenatal? Don't give up. Try taking it at different times of the day, with your largest meal or shortly before bedtime. Avoid taking it on an empty stomach, since the concentrated iron in prenatal vitamins can cause nausea and upset stomach. You can also experiment with different brands or take children's chewable vitamins and supplement with additional folic acid.

Talk to your doctor if you're having trouble with your prenatal vitamin. He or she may prescribe a different prenatal that's easier to digest.

My Experience

I wasn't passionate about prenatal nutrition until I experienced pregnancy myself. And I certainly wasn't an expert in prenatal nutrition until I experienced it myself.

Because it's hard. It's hard to know what to eat and when to eat it, especially if you aren't feeling well. It's hard to make healthy choices when you're too tired to make dinner. It's hard to avoid that 'pregnancy excuse' when you've given up so many things (wine, sushi, restful nights, abs and zip-up jeans, to name a few) already.

I get it. I've been there.

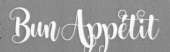

I am there. I'm 30 weeks pregnant with my second child, and healthy eating can still be a daily struggle. Thankfully, perfection is not a prerequisite for pregnancy. What is important is the knowledge that it does matter what you eat during pregnancy (and hopefully you're a believer now!). It also helps to know what to eat and when, and how to help control your appetite and hunger levels.

That's where I can help.

What you'll find in this book

Your baby needs specific nutrients at specific times for optimal growth and development. I'll share what foods contain the nutrients that are so important for baby (and mom!) each trimester. Within each trimester, I've also included two sample meal plans and four recipes with nutrition facts, plus specific weight gain guidelines. Chapter Eight also lists 12 Perfect Pregnancy Snacks that are calorie-controlled, yet sure to satisfy your appetite.

The rest of the book includes guidance on weight gain, controlling appetite and cravings, what to drink and how to prepare for your blood glucose test.

Thank you for allowing me to be your ally on this incredible journey. It's my greatest hope that this book helps to ensure your health and your baby's health and supports the best habits for your growing family.

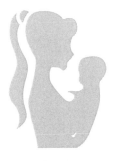

CHAPTER ONE

First Trimester

Your baby grows from
a tiny cluster of cells to...
3 inches long
1 ounce
the size of a lemon

Welcome to pregnancy! The first trimester can be an exciting time, from the first positive pregnancy test to hearing your baby's rapid heart beat for the first time. Some women are fortunate enough to feel fine during the first trimester. If that's not you, fear not. Fatigue, morning sickness (that lasts all day), anxiety and even weight loss are normal occurrences during this phase.

My best advice for healthy eating in the first trimester: Do what you can! Sometimes it's not much, which is why my first trimester recipes are a simple smoothie, easy salad and throw-it-together dinner. Don't be afraid to ask for help with the grocery shopping or to utilize grocery or meal delivery services.

You'll also want to stock up on some easy convenience foods. Load up on healthy staples, such as:

» In the pantry «
Microwavable brown or wild rice
Canned beans
Nuts and nut butter
Low-fat soups
Whole-wheat pasta
Marinara sauce
Tuna packets
Oatmeal
Fortified cereals

» In the freezer «
Frozen chicken breasts
Frozen black bean burgers
Frozen whole-wheat waffles
Frozen edamame
Frozen berries
Veggie steamer bags

Some of your baby's most critical growth happens during the first trimester, so choose the foods that matter most. Make them appetizing in the form of smoothies, shakes, popsicles or soups. Immediately wash and cut your fruits and vegetables when you get home from the store, and place them in clear containers at eye-level in your fridge. You may need quick food options during this trimester to ward off nausea or rapid-onset hunger, so make the easiest choice the nutritious choice.

■ ■ ■

Feeling rotten? An empty stomach is one of the biggest triggers of nausea. Eat something every couple of hours, and choose foods with protein and fiber. These nutrients slow down digestion and keep your stomach feeling full longer. My Perfect Pregnancy Snacks in Chapter Eight provide an ideal combo of protein and fiber.

Ginger is another anti-nausea remedy found in the food aisle. Peel it and crush it like garlic, and add to smoothies, salad dressings, stir-fry or baked goods.

As tempting as they are, try to avoid simple carbs, like chips, candy and baked goods. They're digested rapidly, so they leave your stomach feeling empty again shortly afterwards.

If you're truly struggling to find the will or the way to eat healthy foods (or any foods), try not to worry. This is why a prenatal vitamin is so important, so be sure to take your prenatal every day. Eat when you can. Do your best to make room for the foods listed here.

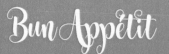

One of the first things to grow in the first trimester – even before your pregnancy test comes back positive – is your baby's neural tube, which includes his or her brain, spinal cord and other tissues of the central nervous system. Much of this growth occurs during the first month of pregnancy, which is why women are advised to take a prenatal vitamin and choose healthy foods while trying to conceive.

Folate is the most critical nutrient for building your baby's neural tube and preventing neural tube defects like spina bifida. It's also essential for making DNA, which is multiplying rapidly right now.

You've probably heard of folic acid. Is it different than folate? Not really. Folate and folic acid are different forms of the same nutrient. Folate comes from food, whereas folic acid is the form found in supplements. Both forms meet your body's needs during this time.

You need 600 micrograms (mcg) of folate per day.

Best food sources of folate

FOOD	AMOUNT
1 prenatal vitamin	400-800 mcg
½ cup cooked spinach	131 mcg
1 serving breakfast cereal, fortified with folate	100 mcg
4 spears cooked asparagus	89 mcg
½ cup cooked Brussels sprouts	78 mcg

Choline also helps to reduce the risk of neural tube defects and promotes brain development in your future baby Einstein.

You need 450 milligrams (mg) of choline per day.

Best food sources of choline

FOOD	AMOUNT
3 ounces beef	356 mg
1 large egg	135 mg
½ cup chickpeas (garbanzo beans)	99 mg
½ cup navy beans	90 mg
¾ cup cooked cauliflower	62 mg
1 cup cooked Brussels sprouts	62 mg
2 Tablespoons wheat germ	21 mg

Iodine is another nutrient that aids spinal cord and brain development. It's also critical for keeping *your* thyroid healthy enough for two during the first trimester. Your baby relies on your thyroid hormone supply until his or her thyroid begins to function on its own, around the beginning of the second trimester.

You need 220 micrograms (mcg) of iodine per day.

Best food sources of iodine

FOOD	AMOUNT
1 gram seaweed	16-600 mcg (varies considerably by source)
3 ounces baked cod	99 mcg
1 cup plain low-fat yogurt	75 mcg
¼ teaspoon iodized salt	71 mcg
1 cup reduced fat milk	56 mcg

Bun Appétit

Another building block for DNA is **zinc**, which is associated with brain and organ development. It also helps your baby's pancreas produce its own insulin starting at the end of the first trimester.

Studies in animals have shown a link between low zinc status during pregnancy and impaired learning and memory later in life. While these studies haven't been done in humans (for good reason!), we know that eating foods rich in zinc can support the health of your baby's growing brain. And that's a no-brainer!

You need 11 milligrams (mg) of zinc per day.

Best food sources of zinc

FOOD	AMOUNT
3 ounces cooked oysters	74 mg
3 ounces beef chuck roast	7 mg
1 serving breakfast cereal, fortified with zinc	4 mg
3 ounces pork chop	3 mg
½ cup canned baked beans	3 mg
1 cup low-fat yogurt	2 mg

First Trimester Weight Gain

In most cases, no weight gain is recommended during the first trimester. See Chapter Six for tips to control your appetite and minimize weight gain.

First Trimester Sample Meal Plan #1

BREAKFAST	Scrambled eggs with a dash of iodized salt Two pieces of whole-wheat toast Two clementines
MID-MORNING SNACK	**Mango Mama-To-Be Smoothie (RECIPE)**
LUNCH	**Mama Caesar Salad (RECIPE)** Baked chips
AFTERNOON SNACK	Half an avocado with cottage cheese
DINNER	Easy dinner platter with **Chipotle Spinach Chips (RECIPE)**, cheese, grapes, bell peppers, hummus, whole-grain crackers and hard-boiled eggs

First Trimester Sample Meal Plan #2

BREAKFAST	Bowl of fortified cereal (like toasted oats, Cheerios, bran flakes, wheat Chex or shredded wheat) Reduced-fat milk Sliced strawberries
MID-MORNING SNACK	Apple with peanut butter
LUNCH	Quinoa bowl with veggies, chickpeas, hard-boiled egg and walnuts Pretzels with hummus
AFTERNOON SNACK	Kiwi and pistachios
DINNER	Leafy green salad with bell peppers, tomatoes, kidney beans and goat cheese topped with **Team Green Goddess Dressing (RECIPE)** Two pieces of dark chocolate

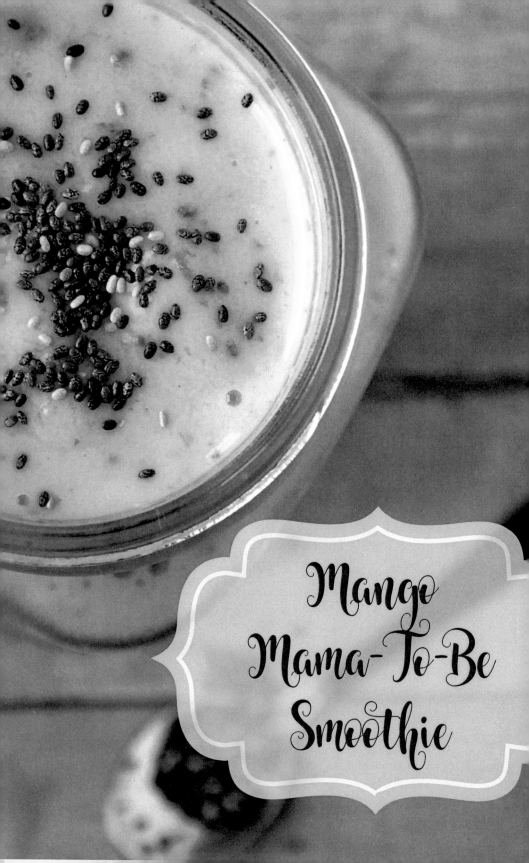

Mango
Mama-To-Be
Smoothie

Smoothies are an easy and delicious way to add more nutrition to your day. This smoothie has folate, calcium, iron and enough fiber and protein to act as an entire meal. It also exceeds your recommended daily intake of vitamin C, which boosts iron absorption and builds baby's bones.

Ingredients

½ cup vanilla Greek yogurt
1 cup frozen mango
½ cup frozen strawberries
1 cup raw spinach
2 dates, pitted
2 teaspoons chia seeds
1 cup cold water

Directions

1. Blend all ingredients together until smooth.

One 18 ounce smoothie contains:

Calories	Fat	Saturated Fat	Total Carbs	Fiber	Protein
338	4g	0.5g	68g	11g	14g

Calcium	Folate	Zinc	Iron	Vitamin C
26%	26%	7%	10%	134%

Percentage of your daily pregnancy needs

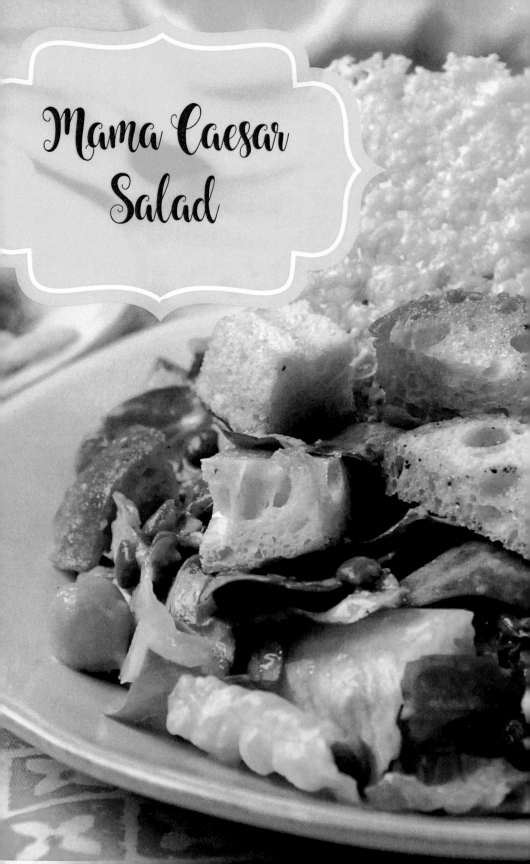

Mama Caesar Salad

Makes 2 large salads
Prep time: 10 minutes

If you love Caesar salad but not the raw eggs or anchovies, here's a pregnancy-safe version that's packed with folate, vitamin C, zinc, iron and calcium.

Ingredients

1 head Romaine lettuce, washed and chopped
2 cups spinach leaves, washed and chopped
8 ounces garbanzo beans
4 ounces lentils
2 Tablespoons Parmesan cheese (optional)

For the dressing:
2 Tablespoons extra virgin olive oil
2 Tablespoons light mayonnaise
2 garlic cloves, peeled
Juice of 1 lemon
½ teaspoon ground yellow mustard
½ teaspoon iodized salt

Directions

1. Mix lettuce, spinach, beans and lentils in a large salad bowl. Set aside.

2. To make dressing, combine olive oil, mayonnaise, garlic cloves, lemon juice, ground mustard and salt in a food processor. Blend until smooth.

3. Drizzle Caesar dressing over salad greens and beans. Garnish with Parmesan crisps if desired.

To make Parmesan crisps, grate a small pile (about one Tablespoon) of Parmesan cheese on a cookie sheet. Bake at 375°F for 8 minutes or until golden and crispy. Let cool on sheet.

To make your own healthy croutons, cut any whole-grain bread into bite-sized pieces and drizzle with olive oil. Bake at 375°F for 8 minutes or until crispy.

One salad (without cheese or croutons) contains:

Calories	Fat	Saturated Fat	Total Carbs	Fiber	Protein
398	20g	3g	44g	12g	13g

Calcium	Folate	Zinc	Iron	Vitamin C
11%	55%	21%	18%	32%

Percentage of your daily pregnancy needs

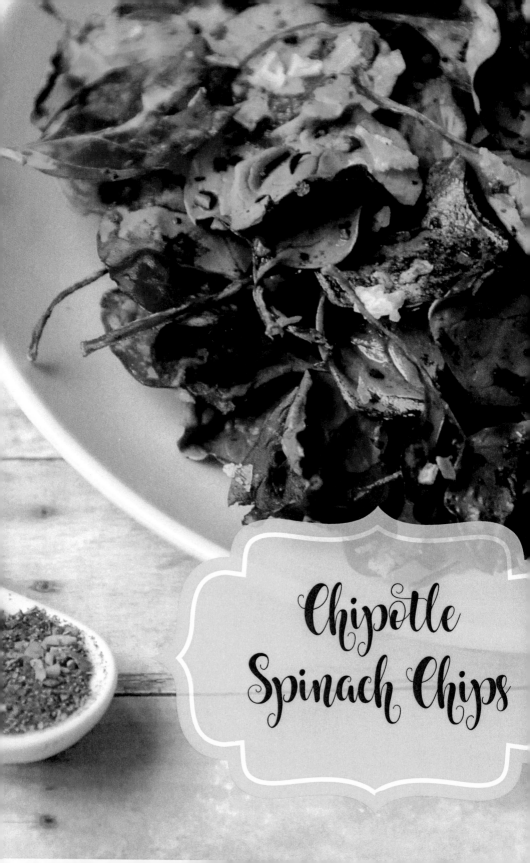

Chipotle
Spinach Chips

Makes 1 cup
Prep time: 3 minutes
Cook time: 15 minutes

You've heard of kale chips. Let me introduce you to spinach chips, which have even more folate than kale, plus loads of other vitamins and minerals. This veggie is perfect for non-salad-lovers and makes a great alternative to potato chips.

Want a dinner that's fast but fancy? Add these to a cutting board along with cheese, grapes, avocado, veggies, hummus, whole-grain crackers and hard-boiled eggs.

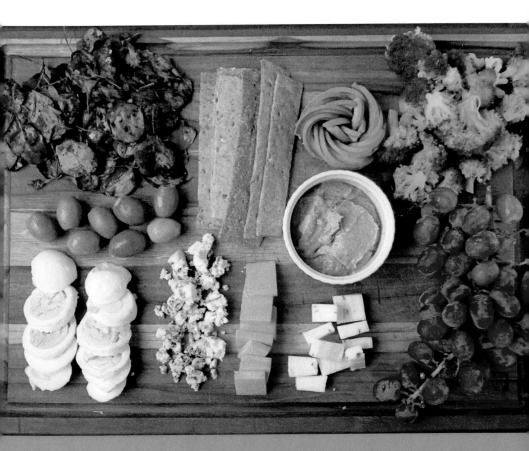

Ingredients

2 cups spinach leaves, washed and patted dry
2 teaspoons extra virgin olive oil
1 teaspoon chipotle powder
½ teaspoon iodized salt
parchment paper

Directions

1. Preheat oven to 275°F. Line two baking sheets with parchment paper.

2. Combine spinach leaves, olive oil and seasonings in a mixing bowl. Mix well.

3. Spread leaves on baking sheets. Avoid overlapping as much as possible.

4. Bake for 15 minutes or until crispy.

A half-cup serving contains:

Calories	Fat	Saturated Fat	Total Carbs	Fiber	Protein
47	5g	0.7g	1g	1g	1g

Calcium	Folate	Zinc	Iron	Vitamin C
3%	10%	1%	3%	10%

Percentage of your daily pregnancy needs

Bun Appétit

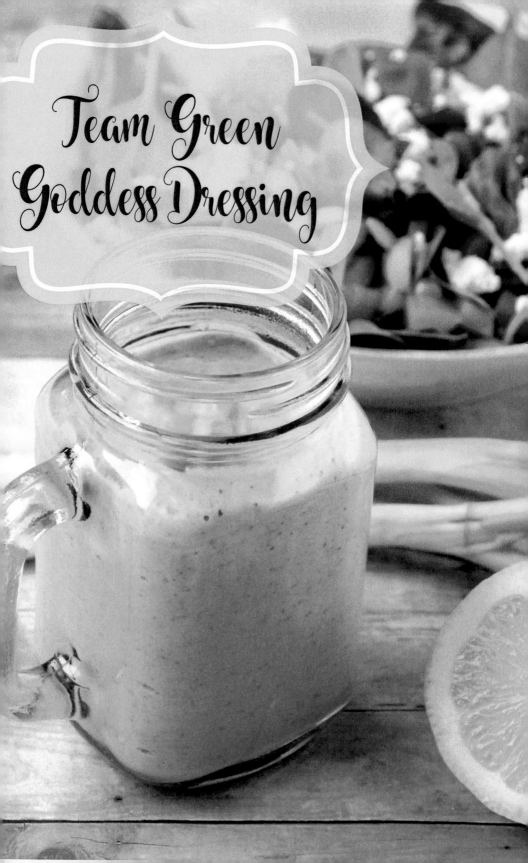

Team Green
Goddess Dressing

Makes 1.5 cups
Prep time: 5 minutes

With spinach, avocado, olive oil and Greek yogurt, this salad dressing qualifies as superfood! Drizzle it over leafy greens with beans and bell peppers to maximize iron absorption. The healthy fats in the dressing also boost antioxidant absorption.

Ingredients

½ cup plain Greek yogurt
1 avocado
2 green onions, chopped (include most of the green shoots)
1 cup spinach leaves
Juice of ½ lemon
1 Tablespoon fresh parsley (or 1 teaspoon dried parsley)
¼ cup fresh basil, loosely packed
3 Tablespoons extra virgin olive oil
2 Tablespoons rice or white wine vinegar

Directions

1. Blend all ingredients together until smooth.

2. Add extra olive oil as needed to thin dressing or reach desired consistency.

A two-Tablespoon serving contains:

Calories	Fat	Saturated Fat	Total Carbs	Fiber	Protein
68	6g	0.9g	3g	1g	1g

Calcium	Folate	Zinc	Iron	Vitamin C
2%	3%	2%	0%	4%

Percentage of your daily pregnancy needs

Second Trimester

Your baby grows from...

2.5-3 inches to 10 inches long

1 ounce to 1-2 pounds

the size of a lemon to

an eggplant

The second trimester may bring some relief from morning sickness, and that crippling fatigue should lessen within a few weeks. You may notice your appetite increasing as you begin to feel better. Or, it may decrease a little if you had a hungry first trimester. Each pregnancy is different, so try not to dwell on every pound gained or lost.

At the beginning of the second trimester, your baby is a fully formed, tiny human being! All of his or her organs, muscles and nerves have developed and are beginning to work as a team. However, there is still plenty of work to be done.

One of the biggest milestones during this period is the growth of your baby's skeleton, which begins turning to bone and will be fully developed by the end of the second trimester. Fingernails and toenails are forming, and vital organs continue to form, mature and start functioning on their own.

Your baby's teeth are also forming underneath the gums. While they may not be visible at birth, tiny tooth buds start mineralizing and building their structure during the second trimester.

Calcium is one of the most critical nutrients for building your baby's bones and teeth, and it keeps your bones strong to carry the extra load of pregnancy.

Baby takes his or her calcium directly from mom's supply, so pregnant women must replenish their own calcium stores throughout pregnancy. Need another reason to choose calcium-rich foods? Research has linked mothers' calcium levels at the end of pregnancy to the beginning of natural labor contractions, indicating less need for the induction of labor.

You need 1,000 milligrams (mg) of calcium per day.

Best food sources of calcium

FOOD	AMOUNT
1 cup low-fat yogurt	315-415 mg
1.5 ounces cheese	310-330 mg
1 cup milk	300 mg
1 cup soymilk, fortified with calcium	300 mg
3 ounces salmon	181 mg
1 serving breakfast cereal, fortified with calcium	100-1,000 mg

Your body needs **Vitamin D** to absorb calcium. Vitamin D is also linked to baby's bone development and immune function. Deficient levels are associated with higher rates of Caesarean births and smaller birth weight babies, as well as baby's risk of Type 1 diabetes and multiple sclerosis.

Vitamin D passes through your placenta to the baby, and your level of vitamin D is directly related to your baby's level at birth. Don't stop thinking about vitamin D once your baby arrives, either! It also passes through breast milk, so your baby's vitamin D intake depends on your supply.

Women carrying extra weight may need extra vitamin D, since obesity increases the risk of vitamin D deficiency. I explain this further in Chapter Seven on *Carrying Extra Weight*.

Some foods contain vitamin D, but the primary source is sunlight. Many experts recommend 5-30 minutes of peak sun exposure at least twice a week, while others recommend minimal sun exposure. There is a delicate balance between adequate sunlight and increased risk of skin cancer.

Bun Appétit

Those with limited sun exposure or dark skin pigmentation may want to consider vitamin D supplementation or having your doctor check your levels.

You can increase your vitamin D supply by eating fish, drinking beverages fortified with vitamin D and taking a prenatal vitamin. The prenatal will provide some vitamin D, but don't rely on it to meet all of your needs. Most prenatals have just 400 International Units (IU), which does not reflect the latest recommendations of 600 IU per day.

You need 600 International Units (IU) of vitamin D per day.

Best food sources of vitamin D

FOOD	AMOUNT
1 Tablespoon cod liver oil	1,360 IU
3 ounces salmon	447 IU
1 prenatal vitamin	400 IU
3 ounces canned tuna fish	154 IU
1 cup orange juice, fortified with vitamin D	137 IU
1 cup milk, fortified with vitamin D	115-124 IU

Another milestone that occurs largely in the second trimester is the increase in blood volume. Simply put, you have more blood to supply your baby and your ever-expanding body with the oxygen that it needs.

Iron is the key transportation method of oxygen within your body, and it helps to supply oxygen-rich blood to you and your baby. Because the demand for iron increases so dramatically during pregnancy, it's possible that your iron needs may not be met without supplementation.

Eat foods that are high in iron and continue taking your prenatal vitamin with iron. Most gummy prenatals don't contain iron, so you may have to take separate iron pills to avoid deficiency. Iron deficiency during the first and second trimesters increases the risk of preterm labor, low birth weight babies and even infant mortality.

You need 27 milligrams (mg) of iron per day.

Best food sources of iron

FOOD	AMOUNT
1 serving breakfast cereal, fortified with iron	18 mg
1 cup canned white beans	8 mg
3 ounces dark chocolate	7 mg
½ cup cooked lentils	3 mg
½ cup cooked spinach	3 mg

■ ■ ■

Low on iron? Iron-deficiency anemia is the most common type of anemia during pregnancy. It occurs because you have nearly 50% more blood circulating in your body. Logically, your iron needs also increase 50% during pregnancy.

Your doctor will likely do blood work at the beginning of pregnancy to check your health status, including your iron levels. If they're low or borderline low, your doctor may prescribe an iron supplement or retest you during pregnancy. If you're feeling weak, dizzy or especially tired, tell your doctor so he or she can recheck your iron status.

A good trick to enhance iron absorption is to eat a meal with both iron and **vitamin C**-rich foods. When eaten together, vitamin C boosts iron absorption. It also helps build bone, teeth and blood cells and supports a healthy immune system.

You need 85 milligrams (mg) of vitamin C per day.

Best food sources of vitamin C

FOOD	AMOUNT
½ cup red bell pepper	95 mg
¾ cup orange juice	93 mg
1 medium orange	70 mg
1 medium kiwi	64 mg
½ cup cooked broccoli	51 mg
½ cup strawberries	49 mg

Second Trimester Weight Gain & Calorie Needs

Weight gain recommendations vary based on your pre-pregnancy BMI. These are basic calorie ranges for the second trimester (assuming no weight was gained in the first trimester). See Chapter Six for more helpful weight gain guidelines and tips to control your appetite.

Normal weight (pre-pregnancy BMI of 18.5-24.9)

☑   Eat 385-415 extra calories per day during the second trimester

Overweight (pre-pregnancy BMI of 25-29.9)

☑   Eat 285-315 extra calories per day during the second trimester

Obese (pre-pregnancy BMI of ≥30.0)

☑   Eat 220-250 extra calories per day during the second trimester

BREAKFAST	**Two Egg Frittata Muffins (RECIPE)** Two patties turkey sausage Banana
MID-MORNING SNACK	Cereal trail mix
LUNCH	Grilled chicken wrap with hummus, spinach and tomatoes Cup of broth-based soup Apple
AFTERNOON SNACK	Brown rice cake with peanut butter and honey
DINNER	**Lentil Chili** with Cornbread Muffin **(RECIPE)** Sautéed asparagus Dessert: One **Angel Food Babycake (RECIPE)**

Second Trimester Sample Meal Plan #2

BREAKFAST	English muffin with peanut butter and jelly Orange Glass of skim milk
MID-MORNING SNACK	Cherries and string cheese
LUNCH	Grilled deli turkey sandwich on whole-wheat bread with avocado, cheese, spinach and tomato Baked chips Side of pickle
AFTERNOON SNACK	Hard-boiled egg, grapes and wheat crackers
DINNER	**Pistachio and Goat Cheese-Crusted Salmon (RECIPE)** Brown or wild rice Leafy green salad with olive oil and balsamic dressing

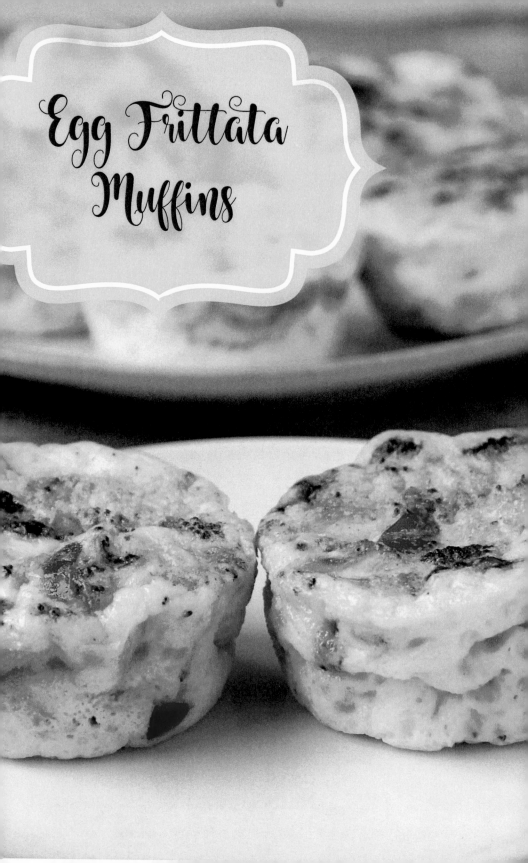

Egg Frittata Muffins

Makes 8 muffins
Prep time: 15 minutes
Cook time: 20 minutes

These muffins can be made ahead of time and stored in the fridge for quick on-the-go breakfasts during the week. Two muffins are rich in vitamin C and a good source of protein, calcium, vitamin D, zinc and folate.

Ingredients

1 cup broccoli, finely chopped
¼ cup bell pepper, finely chopped
¼ cup spinach leaves, finely chopped
1 teaspoon extra virgin olive oil
½ cup whole or reduced fat milk
6 eggs
¼ cup cheddar cheese, shredded
Dash of iodized salt and pepper

Directions

1. Preheat oven to 350°F. Grease muffin tins.

2. Sauté broccoli, bell pepper and spinach in olive oil over medium heat. Cook for 5 minutes or until tender. Remove from heat.

3. In a large liquid measuring cup, combine milk, eggs, cheese and a dash of salt and pepper. Whisk until blended.

4. Add vegetable mixture to muffin cups, dividing evenly among 8 cups.

5. Pour liquid mixture into muffin cups, dividing evenly among 8 cups.

6. Bake for 20 minutes or until toothpick inserted comes out clean. Egg mixture will rise in the oven but return to normal once removed from heat.

7. Serve immediately or store covered in the refrigerator. To reheat muffins, microwave for 20-30 seconds.

Two muffins contain:

Calories	Fat	Saturated Fat	Total Carbs	Fiber	Protein
185	12g	5g	4g	1g	14g

Calcium	Folate	Zinc	Iron	Vitamin C	Vitamin D
15%	11%	13%	7%	39%	12%

Percentage of your daily pregnancy needs

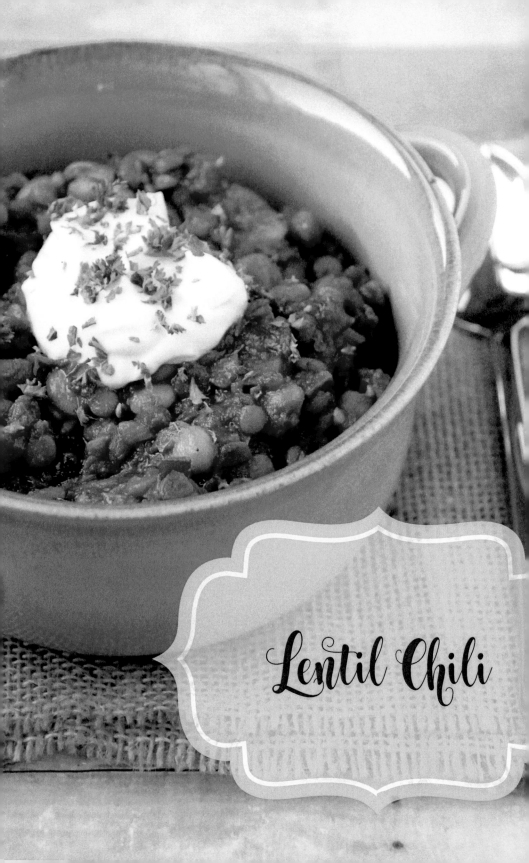

Lentil Chili

Makes 10 cups
Prep time: 15 minutes
Cook time: 35 minutes

This recipe uses canned beans, so your chili can be ready in under an hour! It freezes well, so consider saving half the batch for a delicious, reheat-able meal after baby's arrival. You can also substitute vegetable broth for chicken broth to make this recipe vegan-friendly.

Ingredients

1 cup dried lentils
32 ounces low-sodium chicken or vegetable broth
½ of a white onion, chopped (about 1 cup)
½ of a red bell pepper, chopped (about 1 cup)
1 cup mushrooms, chopped
2 cloves garlic, diced (or 1 teaspoon jarred minced garlic)
1 teaspoon extra virgin olive oil
Two 15 ounce cans pinto beans, drained and rinsed
15 ounce can black beans, drained and rinsed
Two 15 ounce cans diced tomatoes with jalapenos, drained
6 ounces tomato paste
1 Tablespoon chili powder
½ Tablespoon ground cumin

Directions

1. Add lentils and chicken broth to a Dutch oven or large cooking pot. Simmer at medium-low heat for 20 minutes or until lentils are tender.

2. In a separate saucepan, sauté onions and garlic in olive oil for 5 minutes or until onions are translucent. Add to lentils.

3. Add raw bell pepper, raw mushrooms, beans, canned tomatoes, tomato paste, chili powder and cumin to pot with lentils. Mix well and cook on medium heat 10-20 minutes or until heated through.

4. Serve with plain Greek yogurt (a high-protein substitute for sour cream!) or avocado for extra creaminess.

One 1.5 cup serving contains:

Calories	Fat	Saturated Fat	Total Carbs	Fiber	Protein
359	3g	1g	63g	23g	23g

Calcium	Folate	Zinc	Iron	Vitamin C
14%	44%	28%	26%	38%

Percentage of your daily pregnancy needs

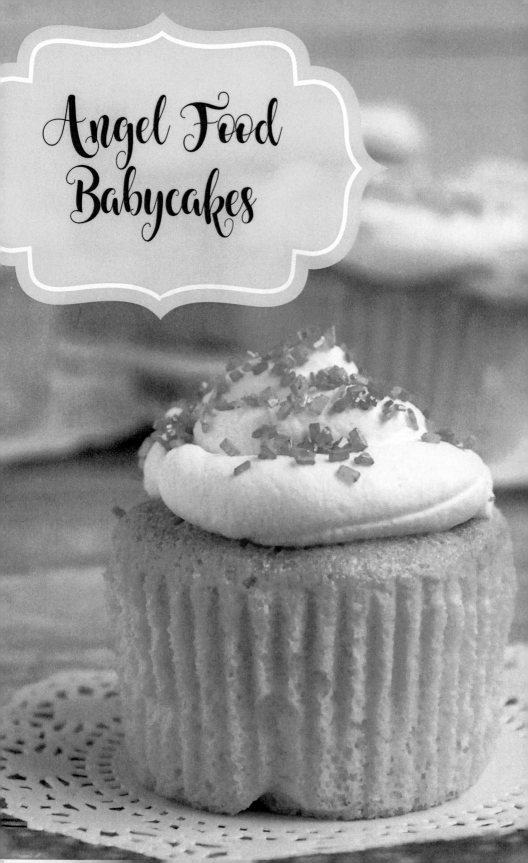

Angel Food Babycakes

Makes 15 cupcakes
Prep time: 25 minutes
Cook time: 20 minutes

Angel food cake is one of the lowest-calorie desserts, but these cupcakes will still satisfy any sweet tooth! Pair with a dollop of whipped cream, strawberries or sprinkles for a dessert fitting of your little angel.

Ingredients

½ cup cake flour
¾ cup powdered sugar (sift before measuring)
¼ teaspoon iodized salt
5 egg whites (or 1 cup liquid egg whites) at room temperature
¾ teaspoon vanilla extract
½ teaspoon cream of tartar
¼ cup granulated sugar

Directions

1. Preheat oven to 350°F.

2. Line muffin tin with 15 cupcake liners. (If your muffin tin holds 12, save 3 liners for a second batch)

3. Sift together cake flour, powdered sugar and salt. Set aside.

4. In a separate mixing bowl, use hand mixer to whisk egg whites on medium speed until very frothy, about 2 minutes.

5. Add vanilla and cream of tartar, beating for another 2 minutes until soft peaks form.

6. Add granulated sugar, one spoonful at a time. Beat between spoonfuls.

7. Beat at medium-high speed until stiff peaks form and batter is shiny, about 5 minutes.

8. Add ¼ of the flour-sugar mixture, folding in with a spatula until incorporated. Continue folding in the remainder in small increments until batter is mixed.

9. Add to cupcake liners, filling to the top.

10. Bake 18-20 minutes or until golden brown and toothpick inserted comes out clean.

One cupcake (without whipped cream) contains:

Calories	Fat	Saturated Fat	Total Carbs	Fiber	Protein
55	0g	0g	12g	0g	2g

Calcium	Folate	Zinc	Iron	Vitamin C
0%	2%	0%	1%	0%

Percentage of your daily pregnancy needs

Bun Appétit

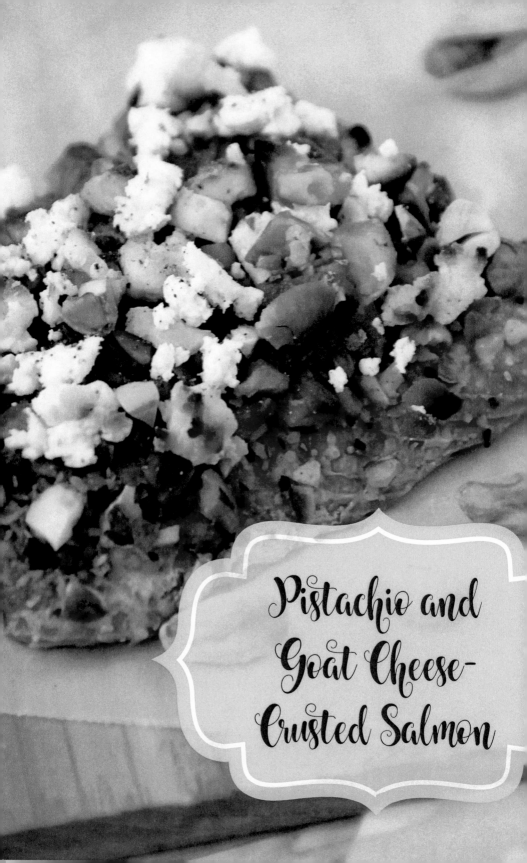

Pistachio and Goat Cheese-Crusted Salmon

Serves two
Prep time: 5 minutes
Cook time: 12 minutes

Salmon and pistachios are excellent sources of omega-3 fats and protein, which are discussed in the Third Trimester chapter. The other MVP of this meal is vitamin D. A 3-ounce filet of salmon meets 75% of your daily vitamin D needs!

Ingredients

2 filets (3-4 ounces each) of wild salmon
1 teaspoon extra virgin olive oil
2 Tablespoons crumbled goat cheese
¼ cup pistachios, out of shell

Directions

1. Preheat oven to 400°F. Line baking sheet with aluminum foil.
2. Crush shelled pistachios by placing in a plastic sandwich bag and using a fork or meat tenderizer to grind to desired size.
3. Drizzle each filet with olive oil, crushed pistachios and crumbled goat cheese.
4. Bake for 12-15 minutes or until salmon is cooked through. Serve.

Get your grill on! You can also cook salmon filets on cedar planks, set to medium heat, for 12 minutes or until cooked through.

One filet contains:

Calories	Fat	Saturated Fat	Total Carbs	Fiber	Protein
287	18g	4g	4g	2g	26g

Calcium	Folate	Zinc	Iron	Vitamin C	Vitamin D
5%	6%	10%	6%	1%	75%

Percentage of your daily pregnancy needs

Third Trimester

Your baby grows from...
10 inches to 18-22 inches long
1-2 pounds to 6-10 pounds
the size of an eggplant to
a small pumpkin

Only a few more weeks until you meet your baby boy or baby girl. It may feel like an eternity still, as third trimester carries on. That first trimester fatigue may be returning, along with some new symptoms like swollen feet, an achy back, heart burn and shortness of breath. Take heart, mamas...you're in the home stretch!

Your third trimester may begin with a blood glucose check at your doctor's office. I've included some tips and sample meals in Chapter Five so you know what to eat – and what to avoid – to improve your chances of passing the test.

The third trimester is the "growth trimester." Your baby has successfully developed most of his or her organs and critical systems by now. The last three months are focused on growth and fat accumulation so your baby will be a chubby cherub by delivery.

Protein is essential for proper growth, so give extra preference to protein-rich foods this trimester. Protein helps keep you feeling full, so it's an important tool in controlling cravings and keeping your weight gain in check. It also helps lessen blood sugar spikes, which makes it especially valuable for anyone monitoring their blood sugar levels.

Aim for at least one source of protein at every meal, and protein with every snack, to support your baby's growth.

Protein needs vary based on an individual's body weight and activity level. Aim for at least 65-75 grams (g) per day during pregnancy.

Best food sources of protein

FOOD	AMOUNT
3 ounces chicken breast	26 g
3 slices deli turkey breast	18 g
3 ounces salmon	17 g
½ cup cottage cheese	14 g
½ cup cooked lentils	9 g
½ cup canned kidney beans	8 g
1 cup milk	8 g
2 Tablespoons peanut butter	8 g
1 egg	6 g

Third trimester is the ideal time to eat **prebiotics** and **probiotics**. Prebiotics, found in most fruits and vegetables, nourish the healthy bacteria in your gut.

Probiotics *are* the good bacteria, which support intestinal health and discourage the growth of disease-causing bacteria. In adults, healthy gut bacteria are linked to weight control, reduced inflammation, bowel regularity and reduced risk of chronic diseases.

It was originally believed that babies were born with a sterile gut, or a "bacteria blank slate," until their trip through the birth canal. Now there is evidence that your diet directly affects the gut bacteria found in your placenta, which transfers nutrients to baby. In other words, the beneficial prebiotics and probiotics you eat now are indeed passed on to your baby, in one form or another. Once your baby is born, breast milk will become his or her biggest source of healthy bacteria.

There is currently no formal recommended daily allowance of prebiotics or probiotics.

Best food sources of prebiotics

Fruits and vegetables, especially bananas, asparagus and artichokes

Garlic, leeks and onions

Whole grains

Best food sources of probiotics

Yogurt with live cultures

Sourdough bread

Kefir

Sauerkraut

Tempeh (fermented soybeans)

Miso soup

"Eating for two" is a myth, but you should be drinking for two. Staying hydrated can reduce the risk of many pregnancy complications, like preterm labor, preeclampsia and low amniotic fluid. Check Chapter Four for more about fluids and advice on what to drink if you don't love water. I also reveal the verdict on diet sodas, tea and artificial sweeteners during pregnancy.

At a minimum, you need three Liters of **fluid**, or nearly 13 cups, per day during this stage of pregnancy. That includes fluids from all sources, including foods, fruits, smoothies, milk with your cereal and so on.

Keep in mind that there's a delay in our bodies' thirst signals. If you're feeling thirsty, your body is already somewhat dehydrated. Don't wait for thirst as a reminder to stay hydrated. Be proactive about drinking fluids throughout the day, even if you have to set reminders for yourself or carry a water bottle at all times. And if you're not a water-lover, rest assured that there are plenty of alternative flavored beverages to keep you sipping away.

Fluid needs vary based on many factors, including an individual's body weight and activity level. Aim for at least 3 Liters of fluid per day during pregnancy.

Best sources of fluids

Water
Flavored water
Milk
Light fruit juice
Fruits, soups, gelatin, popsicles and other foods

Some of the most fascinating new research in pregnancy nutrition is on **omega-3 fats**, a type of polyunsaturated fat. They've been linked to many important things in pregnant women, including:

☑ reduced preterm birth in both normal and high-risk pregnancies

☑ greater baby birth weight and head circumference

☑ early visual and brain development in baby

☑ reduced risk of postpartum depression

☑ reduced risk of allergies in infants

Omega-3 fats can help improve pregnancy outcomes and reduce your risk of postpartum depression. They're also considered critical building blocks for baby's brain and eyes. Your baby's brain accelerates its growth during the second half of pregnancy, so it's important to have these nutrients now.

As essential as omega-3 fats are, your body can't make them on its own. They must be consumed in your diet. Unfortunately, the average American diet is severely lacking in omega-3s.

Don't be afraid of eating enough fish during pregnancy. Many women are scared of ingesting harmful levels of mercury, but the greater danger may be eating too little omega-3s from seafood.

The benefits listed above are most commonly seen by eating 1-2 servings of fish per week. This amount is within safe mercury guidelines, so the benefits will far outweigh any risk of mercury overconsumption.

There is currently no formal recommended daily allowance for omega-3 fats. Aim for at least 1 gram (g) per day.

Best food sources of omega-3 fats

FOOD	AMOUNT
1 Tablespoon flaxseed oil	7 g
1 Tablespoon chia seeds	2.5 g
1 ounce walnuts	2.5 g
3 ounces salmon	2.2 g
1 Tablespoon ground flaxseed	1.6 g
1 Tablespoon canola oil	1.3 g
½ cup tofu, firm	733 mg
½ cup edamame	280 mg

■ ■ ■

See DHA on your food label? DHA (docosahexaenoic acid) is a type of omega-3 found most frequently in brain and eye tissues. Your baby starts accumulating DHA in utero, although the amount depends on how much DHA is consumed in the mother's diet. Some foods, like eggs, yogurt, milk and baby formula, are now being fortified with DHA. Check your labels!

Third Trimester Weight Gain & Calorie Needs

Weight gain recommendations vary based on your pre-pregnancy BMI and pregnancy weight gain thus far. These are basic calorie ranges for the third trimester (assuming consistent weight gain during the second trimester and no weight gain in the first trimester). See Chapter Six for more helpful weight gain guidelines and tips to control your appetite.

Normal weight (pre-pregnancy BMI of 18.5-24.9)

☑ Eat 530-560 extra calories per day during the third trimester

Overweight (pre-pregnancy BMI of 25-29.9)

☑ Eat 440-470 extra calories per day during the third trimester

Obese (pre-pregnancy BMI of ≥30.0)

☑ Eat 315-350 extra calories per day during the third trimester

 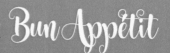

Third Trimester Sample Meal Plan #1

BREAKFAST	Oatmeal with 1 Tbsp peanut butter, nuts, raisins and a sprinkle of brown sugar Banana Glass of skim milk
MID-MORNING SNACK	Almonds and a clementine
LUNCH	**Farro Strawberry Goat Cheese Salad (RECIPE)** Pita bread with hummus Apple
AFTERNOON SNACK	Caprese Snack: Cherry tomatoes and mozzarella balls
DINNER	**3-Ingredient Butternut Squash Soup (RECIPE)** Whole wheat dinner roll Zucchini noodles sautéed in olive oil Dessert: Two pieces dark chocolate

Third Trimester Sample Meal Plan #2

BREAKFAST	Greek yogurt with blueberries ½ Grapefruit Hard-boiled egg Glass of light orange juice
MID-MORNING SNACK	Bell peppers and carrots with hummus
LUNCH	**Chickpea Tahini Bowl (RECIPE)** ½ of grapefruit Iced tea
AFTERNOON SNACK	Chips with salsa and ¼ avocado
DINNER	Whole-wheat pasta with turkey meatballs Steamed broccoli Dessert: One **Ready to Pop-Corn Treat (RECIPE)**

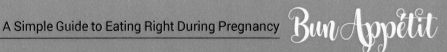

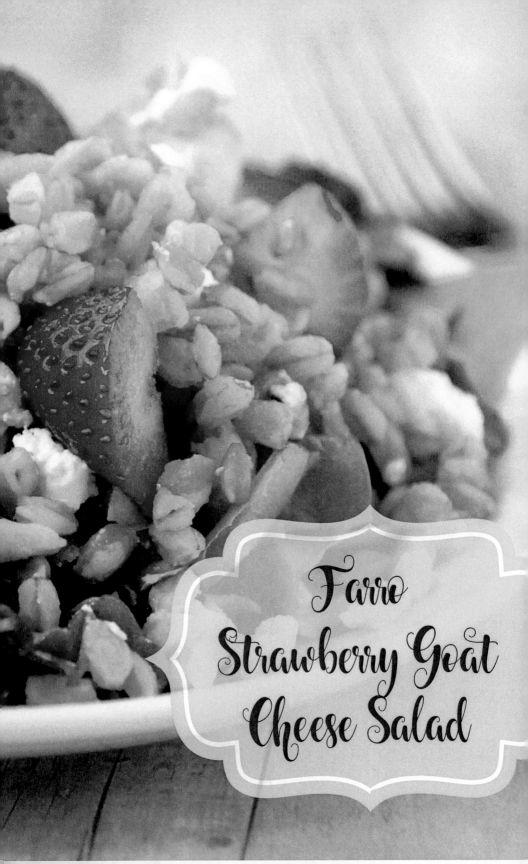

Farro Strawberry Goat Cheese Salad

Serves four
Prep time: 5 minutes
Cook time: 20 minutes

Have you heard of farro? It's an ancient grain with similar nutritional value to quinoa: high in protein, fiber and iron. Add some strawberries and avocado, and their vitamin C boosts the absorption of iron from the farro and spinach.

Ingredients

½ cup dry farro (about 1.5 cups cooked)
1 avocado, sliced into cubes
8-10 strawberries, sliced
¼ cup goat cheese
6 cups spinach leaves
Drizzle of extra virgin olive oil

Directions

1. Cook farro according to package instructions. Dry farro will expand about 3 times its size when cooked. Farro can be served warm or cold.

2. Combine farro, avocado, strawberries and goat cheese in large bowl.

3. Drizzle with olive oil and serve over leafy greens.

One salad contains:

Calories	Fat	Saturated Fat	Total Carbs	Fiber	Protein
239	12g	3g	28g	9g	8g

Calcium	Folate	Zinc	Iron	Vitamin C
9%	23%	6%	10%	49%

Percentage of your daily pregnancy needs

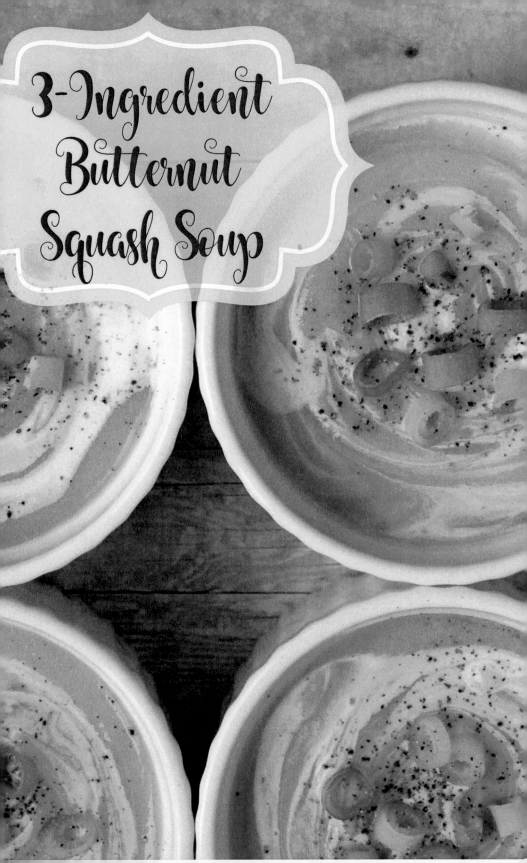

3-Ingredient Butternut Squash Soup

Makes 4.5 cups
Prep time: 5 minutes
Cook time: 50 minutes

With just three ingredients (plus optional garnishes), this is one of the easiest-ever soups. And it's delicious! Cook the butternut squash ahead of time to save yourself time during the week. Just one cup provides more than a full day's worth of vitamin A, which aids baby's growth and development and visual health.

Ingredients

1 butternut squash, washed
16 ounces low-sodium chicken or vegetable broth
¼ cup heavy whipping cream
Black pepper to taste (optional)
Sliced green onion for garnish (optional)

Directions

1. Preheat oven to 350°F. Cut butternut squash in half length-wise and remove inner seeds and pulp. Place halves flesh side down on a cookie sheet.

2. Add a shallow layer of water to the cookie sheet, just enough to cover the bottom of the sheet. Bake for 50 minutes.

3. Place cooked squash and broth in a large blender and puree until smooth.

4. If you're using a high-power blender (like a Vitamix or Blendtec), turn to medium-high speed for 1-2 minutes to heat thoroughly. Otherwise, transfer the soup to a saucepan set at medium-high heat until hot.

5. Serve. Drizzle with heavy whipping cream, divided evenly among four bowls (about 1 Tablespoon per serving).

6. Garnish with black pepper and green onion, as desired.

One cup of soup contains:

Calories	Fat	Saturated Fat	Total Carbs	Fiber	Protein
132	6g	4g	18g	5g	4g

Calcium	Folate	Zinc	Iron	Vitamin C
8%	5%	3%	4%	27%

Percentage of your daily pregnancy needs

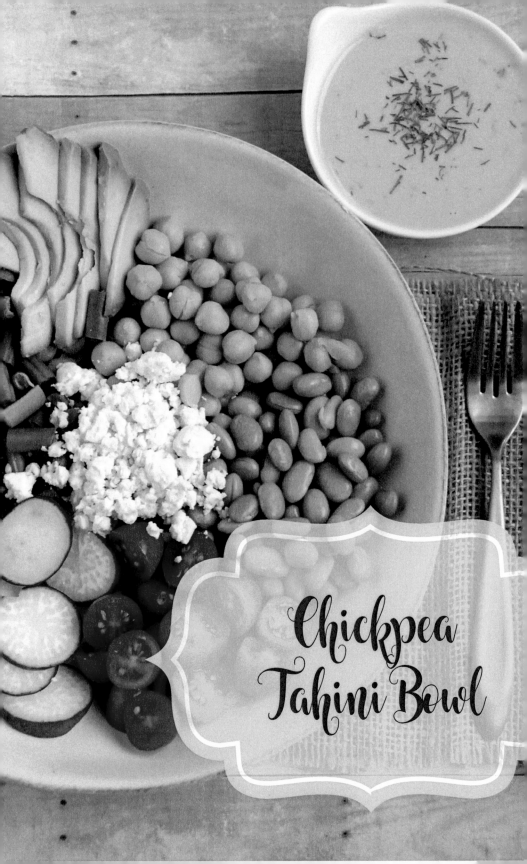

Chickpea
Tahini Bowl

Serves two
Prep time: 15 minutes

Dinner doesn't have to be complicated, especially during the third trimester! This one takes 15 minutes to throw together, and you'll be bowled over by the flavor and nutrient value. It's a good stand-alone dinner, or you can pair with a side of soup, piece of fruit or crusty whole-grain bread.

Ingredients

½ cup chickpeas (a.k.a. garbanzo beans), rinsed
½ cup cherry tomatoes, sliced
½ cup raw green beans, chopped
2 radishes, sliced
½ cup edamame beans (also called mukimame)
½ avocado, sliced
2 Tablespoons pasteurized feta cheese

For the tahini dressing:
½ cup hummus
½ teaspoon extra virgin olive oil
1 garlic clove, minced
Juice from ¼ lemon
½ teaspoon dried dill

Directions

1. Add all dressing ingredients in a small bowl. Mix well.

2. Assemble all other ingredients in a serving bowl. Drizzle with tahini dressing.

One serving contains:

Calories	Fat	Saturated Fat	Total Carbs	Fiber	Protein
328	18g	3g	34g	12g	13g

Calcium	Folate	Zinc	Iron	Vitamin C
11%	39%	25%	14%	25%

Percentage of your daily pregnancy needs

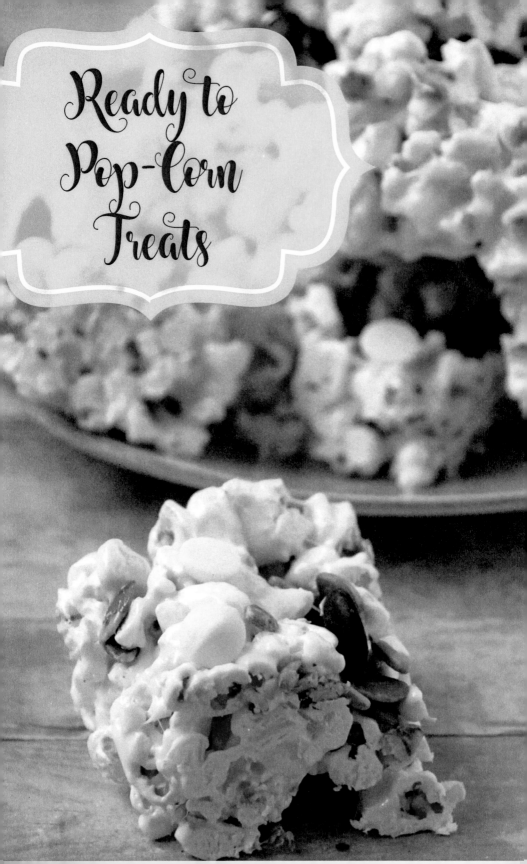

Ready to Pop-Corn Treats

Makes 16 treats
Prep time: 30 minutes

These popcorn treats are a spin off Rice Krispies Treats™ and a healthier homemade substitution for flavored gourmet popcorn. The popcorn provides a bit of whole-grain fiber, and the sunflower and pumpkin seeds boost the beneficial omega-3 fats.

Ingredients

2 Tablespoons butter
10 ounces marshmallows
8 cups popped popcorn, all kernels removed
1 Tablespoon sunflower seeds
3 Tablespoons pumpkin seeds
¼ cup white or dark chocolate chips

Directions

1. Melt butter and marshmallows over medium heat in a large saucepan.

2. Once melted, add popcorn (be sure all un-popped kernels are removed!). Fold and stir until all popcorn pieces are coated with marshmallow mixture.

3. Remove from heat and spread with spatula or wooden spoon into a medium-sized baking dish.

4. Top with sunflower seeds, pumpkin seeds and chocolate chips.

5. Let cool, about one hour. When ready to serve, cut into small pieces using a serrated knife.

One popcorn treat contains:

Calories	Fat	Saturated Fat	Total Carbs	Fiber	Protein
114	4g	2g	20g	1g	2g

Calcium	Folate	Zinc	Iron	Vitamin C
0%	1%	3%	1%	0%

Percentage of your daily pregnancy needs

CHAPTER FOUR

Drinking for Two

What to Drink During Pregnancy?

Staying well hydrated is one of the best things you can do during pregnancy. That's because dehydration is linked to premature labor, preeclampsia and low amniotic fluid levels. It can be difficult for pregnant women to drink enough fluids, due to caffeine restrictions and changes in your taste preferences (not to mention frequent trips to the bathroom!).

What if you don't love the taste of plain water? Rest assured there are still plenty of excellent options available.

Flavor water with lemon, citrus or other fruit infusions. Some water bottles make this easy by having separate fruit compartments. Add your favorite fruits or herbs and fill with cold water for a lightly flavored beverage.

Another option is adding liquid flavor enhancements to water. These are low in calories but can turn your plain water into strawberry lemonade, fruit punch, peach tea or mango passion fruit, to name a few. They contain small amounts of artificial sweeteners like sucralose and acesulfame-K, but these sweeteners have been deemed safe during pregnancy by the Food and Drug Administration (FDA). You may want to avoid or limit the flavor enhancers with caffeine, however.

You can opt for light fruit juice, or 100% fruit juice cut with water to reduce the sugar load.

Skim or reduced fat milk is a good source of protein, calcium and vitamin D during pregnancy. If you're dairy intolerant, soy milk is most similar to cow's milk, nutritionally speaking. Choose soy milk that has been fortified with calcium and vitamin D. Surprisingly, almond milk is very low in protein, and homemade versions are low in calcium, as well.

Is diet soda safe?

I have a confession. It was during my first pregnancy that I *started* drinking diet soda (non-caffeinated). It's often vilified in the media because of a few misinterpreted "bad science" research studies. Hundreds of studies and decades of research have established the safety of drinking one or two diet sodas per day. There's no reason pregnant women need to avoid diet sodas, but stick with non-caffeinated varieties and be sure to include a variety of fluids in your diet.

I've had some clients complain that diet sodas cause headaches for them. Other pregnant women use soda to relieve nasty headaches, which can be helpful when pain-relief medications are restricted. The answer here may be different for everyone, so listen to your body. If you believe headaches or other negative symptoms are related to diet sodas, they may not be a healthy choice for you.

What about tea?

There is ongoing debate about the safety of drinking tea during pregnancy. The FDA does not regulate herbs, so herbal teas are not FDA-approved during pregnancy. Most non-herbal teas contain caffeine, which should be limited during pregnancy.

The bottom line is to practice moderation; one or two cups of tea per week shouldn't lead to health problems. If you're drinking more than that, talk to your doctor about which teas are safe to drink.

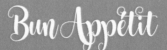

And alcohol?

According to the American Academy of Pediatrics, no amount of alcohol is considered safe to drink during any trimester of pregnancy. Obstetricians have varying views on this topic, so talk to your doctor to get his or her professional opinion.

Read on for a Watermelon Ginger Martini "mocktail" that's perfectly safe during pregnancy.

Watermelon Ginger Martini "Mocktail"

Serves two
Prep time: 5 minutes

This mocktail is fruity and refreshing, and the ginger can help relieve nausea. You can find ginger in your grocery store's produce section, usually near the garlic. Wash, peel or cut off the skin and use a garlic press to extract the ginger's juice. Serve in a martini glass for full effect!

Want a sweet dessert? Substitute frozen watermelon (or any frozen fruit) for the watermelon to create a mouthwatering slushie.

Ingredients

1 cup watermelon, cubed
½ cup cold water
Juice of ½ lemon
Juice of small piece of ginger, about the size of a dice
½ teaspoon Stevia baking powder (optional, for added sweetness)

Directions

1. Add watermelon and water to blender or food processor.

2. Add lemon juice and juice of ginger using a garlic press or citrus hand-squeezer

3. Add sweetener, if desired

4. Process until smooth, about 15 seconds. Serve.

One mocktail contains:

Calories	Fat	Saturated Fat	Total Carbs	Fiber	Protein
25	0g	0g	7g	1g	0.5g

Calcium	Folate	Zinc	Iron	Vitamin C
0%	0%	0%	0%	13%

Percentage of your daily pregnancy needs

CHAPTER FIVE

The Glucose Test

What to Eat to Minimize Your Chances of Gestational Diabetes

The glucose test is a rite of passage into the third trimester and a source of great worry for many women. Here's an overview of what to eat - and what not to eat - to give you the best possible chance of a positive experience (and a negative test result!).

Please note that these suggestions are for the standard blood glucose test given by many obstetricians and should not take the place of detailed instructions given by your doctor. Blood glucose tests have different pre-requisites, so follow the advice of your physician first.

For a standard blood glucose test, here's:

What to Eat:

☑ A balanced meal with whole grains, protein and/or healthy fats **approximately 3 hours before your test**

☑ Water at any time leading up to your test

What Not to Eat:

☑ **Any food** within 2 hours of the test, including Life Savers, mints and sugared gum

☑ An abnormally large meal with heavy carbohydrates anytime on the day of your test

☑ Coffee within 2 hours of the test

Zero-calorie beverages like diet soda shouldn't affect your test, but stick to water only for the fasting period before your test.

How can I trick the test?

Unfortunately, you can't really 'trick' the glucose test. If your body has developed gestational diabetes, there's not much you can do on test day to hide it.

And that's a good thing, I promise! Babies do not like living in a sugary environment, and complications can result from untreated gestational diabetes. If your body is not processing sugar correctly, you need to know so you can treat it and avoid complications for both yourself and your baby.

Can I mess up the results?

If you don't have gestational diabetes, even a large meal three hours before the test shouldn't skew your results. Your body is that good at handling extra blood sugar.

However, if you eat a huge pasta meal immediately before the test, chances are your blood sugar will still be high even if you don't have gestational diabetes. It takes your body 2-3 hours to normalize high levels of sugar in your blood, which is why these fasting guidelines exist. If you've eaten within 2 hours of your appointment, tell your doctor so you can reschedule the test.

 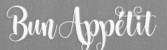

■ ■ ■

Borderline positive for high blood sugar? Your doctor will likely continue testing to determine whether you're making enough insulin to handle the sugar in your food. He or she may prescribe full gestational diabetes protocol, even if your test is borderline or inconclusive. That's because new research shows aggressive treatment to borderline diabetes yields better outcomes for healthy-weight babies (as very large babies can increase birth complications), healthier deliveries, reduced risk of cesarean section and less weight gain in women.

Sample breakfast meals before the glucose test:

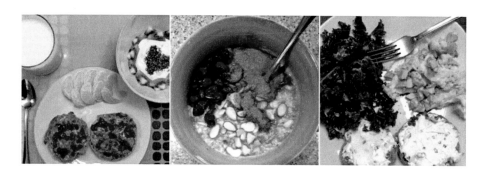

Option A:

Whole-wheat English muffin with peanut butter and jelly
One clementine
Greek yogurt parfait with 1/2 kiwi fruit and chia seeds
Glass of skim milk

Option B:

Oatmeal made with skim milk and drizzled with almonds, dried cranberries and cinnamon

Option C:

Egg scramble with avocado and cheese
Whole-wheat English muffin with cream cheese
Kale salad

Sample lunch meals before the glucose test:

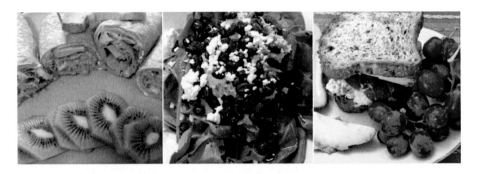

Option A:

Turkey roll-up in whole-wheat wrap with hummus, light mayo, avocado and veggies
One kiwi fruit

Option B:

Spinach salad with tuna packet, black beans, feta cheese and olive oil & balsamic dressing

Option C:

Egg salad sandwich on sprouted grain bread with spinach & avocado
Cluster of grapes
Side of pickle

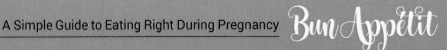

CHAPTER SIX

Weight Gain Guidelines

Tips to Control Your Appetite and Satisfy Your Cravings

I'll be honest. When I was pregnant with my first child, I gained eight pounds in the first trimester. You know...that trimester when you're not supposed to gain any weight. I used my exciting new pregnant status as an excuse to eat anything and everything for a few weeks. When I got to my next checkup, my doctor suggested that I hit the brakes. In her words, "Be sure to leave some pounds to gain at the end of pregnancy, when you'll really need them!"

Even dietitians can get caught up in the 'pregnancy excuse' and struggle to control cravings. The first trimester can feel especially difficult. Your calorie needs haven't changed yet, but junk food sounds most appetizing. And eating frequently helps reduce nausea and fatigue. It's the perfect recipe for gaining a little too much, a little too soon.

In my case, I dropped the pregnancy excuse, got back to my normal eating habits and ultimately gained a healthy amount of weight in 40 weeks.

It's important to reiterate that perfection isn't required during pregnancy. We all make excuses from time to time. I still justify the occasional food choice because I'm pregnant, but it's not every day. Pregnancy shouldn't be a "free pass" to follow your every food whim for 40 weeks.

Here are my tips, both as a professional dietitian and someone who has "been there," to control your appetite and gain weight in a healthy way.

☑ Try not to let pregnancy become an excuse to eat junk. When you hear yourself justifying something "because I'm pregnant," take a pause. It's normal to justify some food choices throughout pregnancy, but don't let your pregnancy become a crutch for the choices you make every day.

- ☑ "Eating for two" is eating too much! Technically, you're eating for 1.05 by the end of pregnancy, when baby is at his or her biggest. You can drink for two, however, since fluid needs increase and hydration is vital during pregnancy.

- ☑ Develop good habits during pregnancy, and they'll help once baby arrives. Not only for childbirth recovery and any future pregnancies, but also in setting a good example for your kids. Eating healthy foods and changing deep-rooted behavior only gets harder with kids, so start following a healthy lifestyle now.

- ☑ Don't give up the exercise. Follow your doctor's instructions first and foremost. But try to stay active, even if it's just a long walk after dinner or taking the stairs over the elevator. Childbirth is a physically demanding event, and being fit can help with the process of labor and delivery. It also aids recovery in the days and weeks following birth.

Here are the recommended weight gain guidelines, per the Institute of Medicine:

PRE-PREGNANCY BMI	RECOMMENDED WEIGHT GAIN DURING PREGNANCY
Underweight (BMI <18.5)	28-40 pounds
Normal weight (BMI 18.5-24.9)	25-30 pounds
Overweight (BMI 25-29.9)	15-25 pounds
Obese (BMI ≥30.0)	11-20 pounds

How many extra calories should I eat?

Here are recommended "extra calorie" ranges for normal, overweight and obese BMI classifications.

Note that these extra calories apply to the second and third trimesters only, when weight gain is expected to occur. They do not account for weight gain already accrued in the first trimester.

Normal weight (pre-pregnancy BMI of 18.5-24.9)

☑ Eat 385-415 extra calories per day during the second trimester

☑ Eat 530-560 extra calories per day during the third trimester

Overweight (pre-pregnancy BMI of 25-29.9)

☑ Eat 285-315 extra calories per day during the second trimester

☑ Eat 440-470 extra calories per day during the third trimester

Obese (pre-pregnancy BMI of ≥30.0)

☑ Eat 220-250 extra calories per day during the second trimester

☑ Eat 315-350 extra calories per day during the third trimester

Please, don't be fooled by these extra calorie allowances! They don't go quite as far as you think. It's one extra muffin per day…or one avocado… or a slightly larger helping at dinner…or 1-2 of my Perfect Pregnancy Snacks at 200-calories apiece (see Chapter Eight). The majority of these "bonus calories" should come from healthy, nutrient-rich foods to nourish your growing baby and build your own nutritional stores.

Also, these are basic suggestions only. Please work with your doctor or a registered dietitian to customize total daily caloric intake specifically for you.

Tips to Control Your Appetite and Satisfy Your Cravings

☑ Improve your mindfulness at mealtimes. Turn off the TV and put away your phone to reduce common distractions that lead to overeating. Slow down, sit down and eat at a table. Focus on the food in front of you, and listen to your body's fullness signals.

☑ Never allow yourself to get too hungry. Feeling starving often leads to less healthy food choices, particularly comfort foods high in fat and sugar, and overeating. Curb your hunger by eating smaller meals consistently throughout the day and planning between-meal snacks with protein and fiber.

☑ Focus on what foods to add, rather than what foods to avoid. Fruits and vegetables should make up nearly half of what we eat, and these fiber-rich foods help satisfy hunger and may naturally decrease portion sizes elsewhere.

☑ Reserve dining out and takeout for special occasions only. Preparing meals at home keeps you in control of the ingredients and can save hundreds of calories per meal.

☑ Don't leave cookies on the counter! Research links food visibility to higher levels of hunger, salivation and consumption. Stash the treat foods out of sight and out of mind, and keep healthier foods more visible.

☑ In the fridge, place your fruits and veggies at eye level in a clear bowl or plastic container. This increases the likelihood that you'll reach for them when you open the fridge. We all stand in front of the fridge looking for something to eat, so make the healthy choice the easiest choice.

 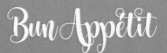

☑ Follow the same rule in the pantry: place the healthiest foods at eye level. Keep your nuts, whole grains, dried fruit and oatmeal in the VIP section. You can also prepare individual grab-and-go snack bags for when you're in a rush or want automatic portion control. Good choices are homemade trail mix, dried cereal, whole-grain crackers and nuts.

☑ Use the freezer for food storage. This works for chocolate, candy, nuts, muffins, cookies and cakes – many of the foods that can be hard to stop once you start. Storing them in the freezer keeps them out of sight and forces you to slow down while you're eating, or wait until it thaws altogether. Eating slowly will make you more mindful of your body's fullness cues. And waiting even a few minutes may help the cravings pass, especially if you drink a glass of water, nosh on something healthier or get occupied doing something else.

☑ Do a little food prep. Wash and slice your veggies so they're easy to grab or add to dinner mid-week. Hard-boil some eggs and cook chicken breasts, quinoa or brown rice for easy meal-starters during the week.

☑ Carry a water bottle everywhere. Our bodies' thirst signals are very similar to our hunger signals. People often mistake these thirst signals for wanting to eat. If you're feeling hungry, drink 1-2 cups of water or flavored water. If you're still hungry 5 minutes later, it's probably true hunger.

☑ We also feel hungry when we're tired. When you can, grab a nap or go to bed before reaching for food. If you're at work, take a short break to walk around or talk to a colleague. And make nighttime sleep a priority: aim for at least 7-8 hours of sleep every night.

☑ Un-super-size your desserts. Serve dessert in a small ramekin, since the smaller dish can help your portion appear larger. Limit the desserts you keep in the house, and instead go out to ice cream as a family once a week. Another approach is having desserts at home that you only "kind of" like. Not a huge fan of mint? Mint ice cream or frozen Peppermint Patties may be just enough to satisfy your sweet tooth without making you crave more.

CHAPTER SEVEN

Carrying Extra Weight

Controlling Weight
Gain If You're Already
Overweight

If you're carrying a few extra pounds into pregnancy, try not to stress about it. Being overweight or obese increases your risk of pregnancy complications, but controlling your weight gain during pregnancy is even more important.

Many of the negative aspects of an overweight pregnancy can be managed with lifestyle factors...factors that are within your control right now.

Stay active, take a prenatal multi-vitamin and watch your portion sizes. Focus on what foods you *should* be eating – those with fiber, lean protein and healthy fats - to keep your appetite under control. Use my tips from Chapter Six, as well as the sample meal plans and snacks included in this book, to limit weight gain to the recommended amounts.

One special consideration for "more to love" mamas

Vitamin D deficiency is more common in people who are overweight. This is because vitamin D is fat-soluble, meaning it gets stored in fat tissues. Once there, it becomes 'trapped' and cannot be used as efficiently by the body.

Many obstetricians in other parts of the world recommend higher intakes of vitamin D during pregnancy for larger women. However, the United States has not changed its daily vitamin D recommendation based on weight, yet.

Your doctor can test for Vitamin D deficiency. If your levels are low, you may need to add a vitamin D supplement or eat more foods rich in or fortified with vitamin D.

CHAPTER EIGHT

Perfect Pregnancy Snacks

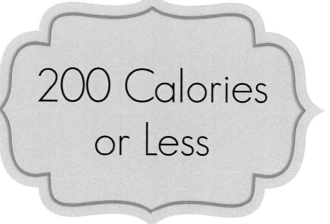

200 Calories or Less

These snacks offer an ideal combination of fiber and protein. Fiber helps to fill you up, whereas protein keeps you feeling full. Plan for 1-2 snacks during the day to keep up with your increasing appetite and control pregnancy cravings.

Each of these snacks is 200 calories or less. By adding one or two of these snacks to your diet every day, you'll meet your extra pregnancy calorie needs. You'll also be feeding your body and your baby with the best nutrients.

I've assembled a dozen quick and easy options that are perfect for spontaneous hunger strikes or when you're feeling tired. They're not just pregnancy snacks, either! Reference this list when you're breastfeeding, looking for healthy toddler snack ideas or anytime you want something convenient, calorie-controlled and dietitian-approved.

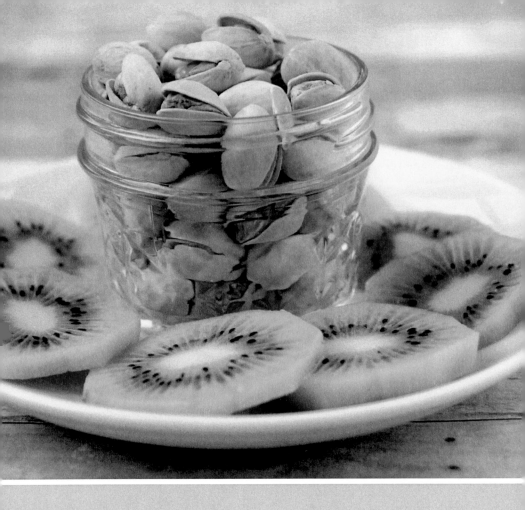

INGREDIENTS:

½ cup pistachios

1 kiwi

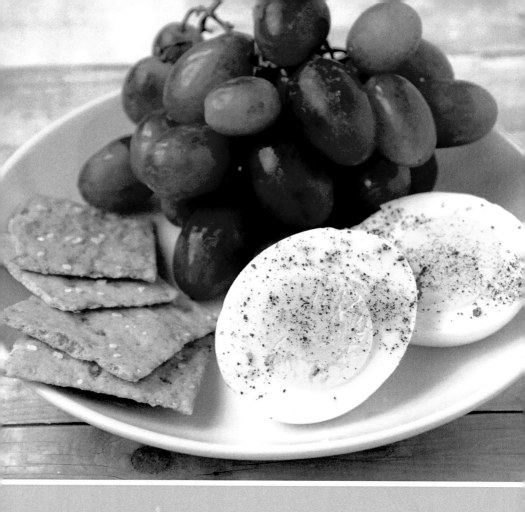

INGREDIENTS:

1 cup grapes

3-4 wheat crackers

1 hard-boiled egg

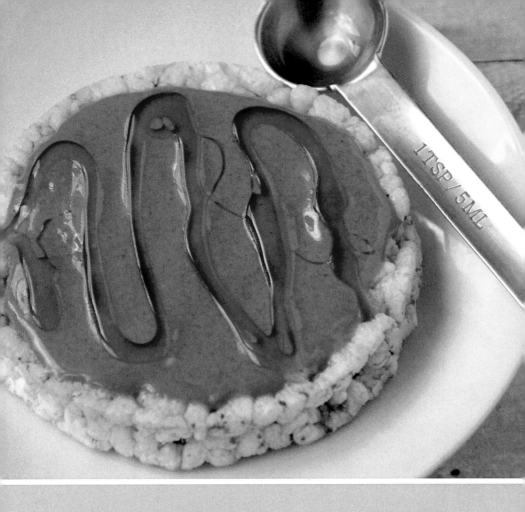

INGREDIENTS:

Brown rice cake

1 Tablespoon peanut butter

1 teaspoon honey

Bun Appétit

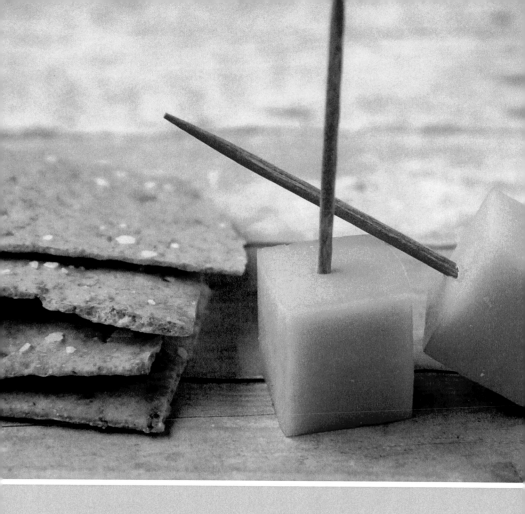

INGREDIENTS:

3-4 wheat crackers

2 cubes cheddar cheese

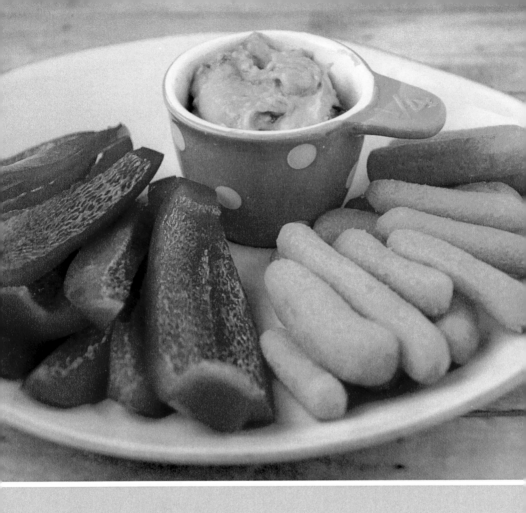

INGREDIENTS:

16 baby carrots

1 cup sliced bell peppers

3 Tablespoons hummus

A Simple Guide to Eating Right During Pregnancy

Bun Appétit

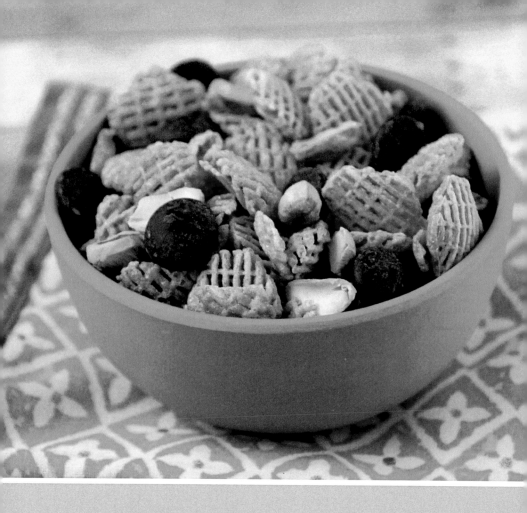

INGREDIENTS:

Trail Mix:

1 cup fortified cereal

10 pistachios

10 chocolate chips

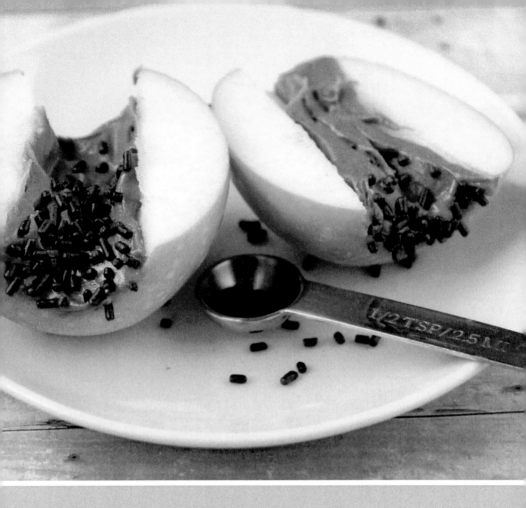

INGREDIENTS:

1 apple

1 Tablespoon peanut butter

½ teaspoon chocolate sprinkles

Bun Appétit

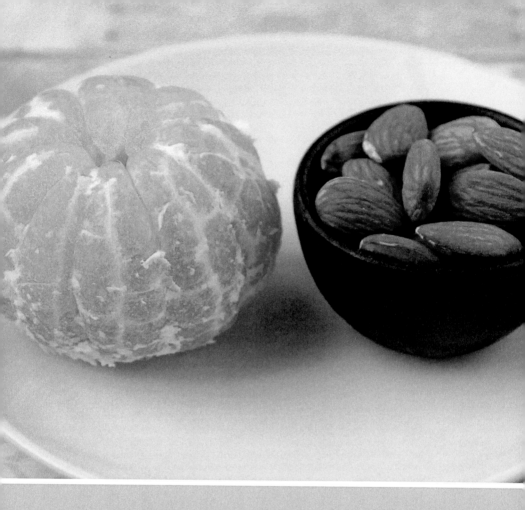

INGREDIENTS:

Mandarin orange

23 almonds

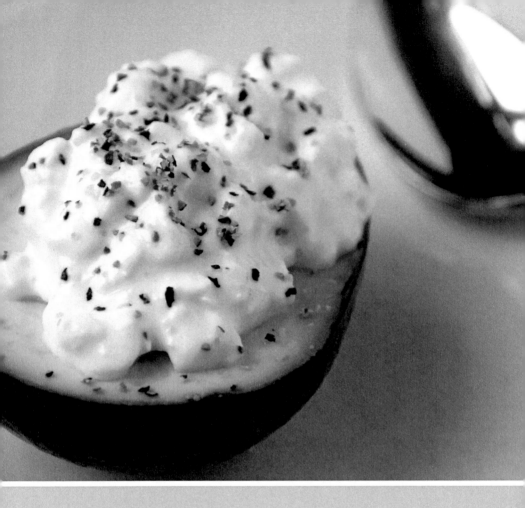

INGREDIENTS:

½ avocado

2 Tablespoons cottage cheese

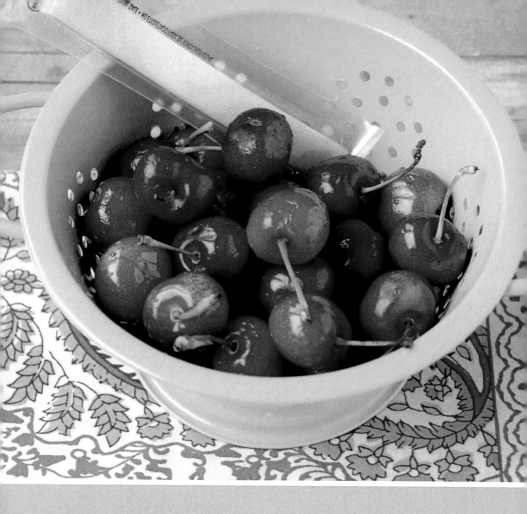

INGREDIENTS:

2 cups cherries

1 string cheese

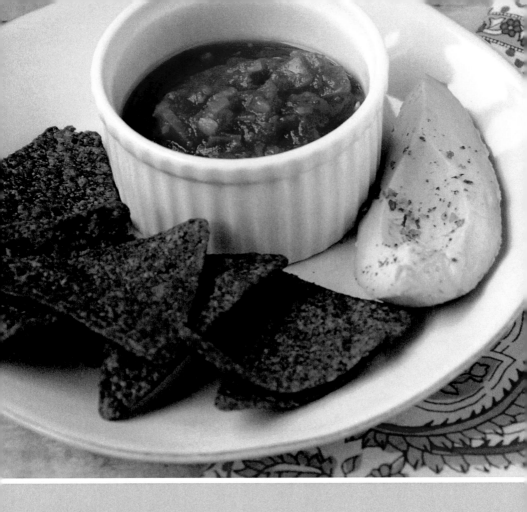

INGREDIENTS:

8 tortilla chips

¼ cup salsa

¼ avocado

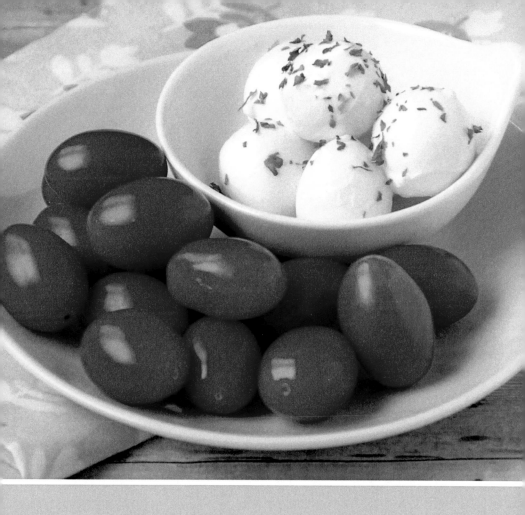

INGREDIENTS:

Caprese Snack:

15 cherry tomatoes

6 mozzarella balls

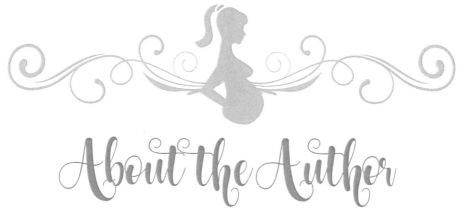

About the Author

Torey Armul is a registered dietitian nutritionist specializing in prenatal and family nutrition, sports nutrition, gastrointestinal diseases and mindful eating. She provides nutrition counseling and corporate consulting services through her private practice, Torey Armul Nutrition.

Torey is a nationally recognized media expert and frequent media contributor. Her expertise is regularly featured in WebMD, U.S. News & World Report, Fox News, Today.com, Shape magazine, Prevention magazine, Fit Pregnancy, Real Simple, MSN.com, Yahoo! and more.

She writes a blog called Best Little Nest with easy recipes, kid-friendly snacks, healthy homemaking tips, crafts, DIY projects and her own experiences in pregnancy and motherhood. Read more at www. BestLittleNest.com.

Torey lives in Columbus, Ohio, with her husband, toddler son and dog. They are adding another baby boy to the nest in February 2017.